The Anabolic Nutrition Program

Dietary Secrets to Gaining Muscle

By Bob Myhal

MuscleMaster.com, Inc.

The Anabolic Nutrition Program
Dietary Secrets to Gaining Muscle

By Bob Myhal

Published by:

MuscleMaster.com, Inc.
153 Northboro Road, Suite 15
Southborough, Massachusetts 01772 U.S.A.

All rights reserved. No part of this publication may be reproduced, stored in a retrieval system, or transmitted, in any form or by any means, electronic, mechanical, photocopying, recording, or otherwise, without prior written permission of Bob Myhal and MuscleMaster.com, Inc.

Copyright © 2002 by Bob Myhal & MuscleMaster.com, Inc.
First printing 1997. Reprinted in 1998, 1999, 2000

Printed in the United States of America

ISBN 0-9722105-1-2

The Anabolic Nutrition Program is intended for healthy adults, age 18 and over. This book is solely for informational and educational purposes and is not medical advice. Please consult a medical or health professional before you begin any new exercise, nutrition, or supplementation program.

All trademarks, service marks, brand names, and product names are the property of their respective owners. The appearance of such names in this publication does not represent endorsement of this publication or this publication's contents. This publication mentions these names solely for informational purposes.

Figures used throughout the text and in charts are for informational purposes only and are believed but not guaranteed to be accurate. This publication is not a substitute for health advice. Readers should seek their physician's advice before acting in reliance upon this publication.

This manual is intended to be accurate and informative; however, there may be errors in content and form. No claim is made that the information contained within is exhaustive. Developing a muscular physique requires a substantial investment of time and effort. Individual results will vary.

You are encouraged to read other available publications and to learn as much as you can on the subject before investing additional time and resources. Neither the author nor MuscleMaster.com, Inc. and its subsidiaries shall have any liability or responsibility to any individual or entity with respect to any loss or damage caused, or alleged to be caused, directly or indirectly by the contents of this publication.

If you wish not to be bound by the above statements, you can return the book to the publisher for a full refund.

Introduction

I'll start by telling you straight-out that the two primary reasons I developed the Anabolic Nutrition Program were frustration and confusion. You see, for years I've been frustrated with the lack of quality nutritional information available for natural athletes looking to add muscle mass.

Sure the muscle magazines always run stories about what some 260 lbs. professional bodybuilder is eating; believe it or not, sometimes it's as much as 9000 calories a day! I even remember reading one article about some behemoth who consumed 5-6 lbs. of beef day in and day out. I'm not kidding. But what this has to do with natural lifters like you and I, individuals who are just looking to pack on some quality muscle mass to look and feel our best, I have no idea.

More recently, in the past 4 or 5 years, a few programs claiming to be geared towards the general fitness population began popping up. At first I was a bit encouraged by this novel trend, but then I actually studied these new programs and even tried most of them out. This is when I became confused.

Not only did a lot of these so-called *muscle building* diet programs blatantly contradict each other—high carbohydrate, low fat; low carbohydrate, high fat; high protein, low carb, low fat; blah, blah, blah—but it also seemed to me that you had to be a chemist to understand them and have a degree in mathematics to make them work.

I'm just trying to add a few pounds of quality muscle mass safely and naturally for crying-out-loud. I don't want to have to change every aspect of my life to accomplish this; and I certainly don't think I need a degree in biochemistry to get the job done.

You see, I have a confession to make: I absolutely detest counting every last calorie. In fact, I just won't do it. Oh sure, I'll make some quick estimates on paper or in my head to give me an idea of where I stand but as for writing every last calorie down and tallying it up, forget about it.

It's not that I'm lazy mind you. I just have plenty of better things to do with my time. And I'm certainly not going to carry a scale and a calculator around with me. That's just not the way I choose to live my life.

Don't get me wrong. This doesn't mean that I'm careless about what I eat or that I'm not in decent shape. It just means that my approach to nutrition is a bit more flexible and realistic than most.

I basically believe that the so-called nutrition experts get way too carried away with numbers and precise details. The human body is a complex machine, I'll give you that, but I don't believe this means a muscle-building nutritional program needs to be overly complex. In fact, I've found that the more complex a diet is, the more difficult it is to stick to it. There is, after all, something to be said for simplicity.

At the same time, we obviously can't just throw anything we want into our bodies. Not if we expect to build a quality, first-rate physique. It just doesn't happen that way.

So with this in mind, I set out to develop an *Anabolic Nutrition Program* not only based in science and the deeply ingrained natural processes of the human body, but also simple to practice and realistic in its expectations. After years of research and extensive experimentation, I've tried just about everything, I've come up with a muscle building diet program that not only works but also is workable.

When you combine this program with quality resistance training, you will add significant muscle mass to your physique. What's more, you won't become a raving, calorie-counting, food-weighing lunatic in the process. This is a good thing.

The bodybuilding lifestyle, after all, should be just a part of a healthy well-rounded physical and intellectual life. It shouldn't be something that we are dominated by. This muscle building diet plan will allow you to pack on the muscle you want to and at the same time still enjoy food and life. This anyway is my goal. I hope it is yours as well.

The nutrition plan itself is broken down into four weeks. While the program will work to take your body through a serious of natural cycles which optimize the release of natural anabolic hormones regardless of what training regimen you follow, I've designed The *Anabolic Nutrition Program* to align perfectly with my 12 Week *Ultimate Muscle Mass Training Program*. Indeed, the two Programs work to complement each other. The 12 Week Training Program matches up with three full cycles of the *Anabolic Nutrition Program* (4 weeks each).

If you haven't tried the *Ultimate Muscle Mass Training Program* yet, I urge you to do so. I doubt that you'll find any better training system for adding muscle safely and naturally. For information about the Program or to order, visit the *Supplement Warehouse* at MuscleMaster.com.

Before we get into the details of *The Anabolic Nutrition Program*, I think it's important to take a brief look at some of the trends in muscle building diet programs as well as some of the more prominent plans currently in vogue.

The Current State of Muscle Building Nutrition

It's important to say right off the bat that when I speak of the "current state of muscle building nutrition" I'm speaking of nutrition as it applies to the natural or drug-free bodybuilder looking to effectively add lean muscle mass.

The natural trainer seeks to gain through healthy nutrition what others might gain from anabolic steroids, synthetic growth hormone, insulin, anticatabolic agents, and a whole array of other often illegal substances. If you've read any of my writing on the subject, you know that for me the legality of these substances is not the entire issue. In general, I don't think the government should be telling adults what they can and cannot put into their bodies, but that's a topic for another occasion.

For me, the issue with these substances is that through various side-effects many of them in some way compromise the user's general health or well-being and thus actually end up working against the healthy lifestyle that I advocate so strongly. But now is not the time nor the place to get too far into this complex and often highly personalized issue. Suffice it to say that for our current purposes we're concerned with nutrition plans that encourage a natural release of muscle building substances and support an all-around healthy lifestyle.

If you know anything about bodybuilding, then you know that the traditional bodybuilding diet has been one that is high in carbohydrates, high in protein, and low in fat.

The carbohydrates, so the reasoning goes, are necessary for energy to fuel intense training sessions. Of course, the need for complex carbohydrates such as whole grains is usually emphasized; the use of simple carbohydrates, most notably processed sugars, is generally restricted or at least discouraged.

An adequate amount of protein is also necessary to build muscle. Through a series of biological processes, proteins, or more specifically the amino acids found in proteins, form the building blocks of muscle tissue. While the specific suggested amounts of daily protein intake varies (more on this later), the importance of a diet high in quality protein sources like lean red meats, fish, skinless chicken and turkey breast, non-fat dairy products, and egg whites has been accepted by the bodybuilding and fitness communities for decades.

As has been mirrored in our society over the past twenty or so years, *fat* in the bodybuilding world has historically been a very bad word. The reasoning goes something like this: if you're trying to develop lean muscle mass, lean being the key word here, then the consumption of fats, particularly saturated fats, will work against this goal. Fat intake, therefore, should be significantly restricted.

Traditionally then, most bodybuilders have stuck to the high carb, high protein, low fat nutritional prescription diligently. The typical daily calorie breakdown using these traditional guidelines would be somewhere in the 65-25-10 range where 65% of the daily calories would be derived from carbohydrates (mostly complex carbs), 25% from protein sources (with the emphasis on low-fat proteins of course), and only 10% from fats (and primarily unsaturated fats). You may have seen some slight flexibility in these numbers from time to time or from program to program, but in general these have been the accepted set-points for individuals looking to add lean muscle mass.

All this should be very familiar to you if you've been training for a while or been watching TV at all in the last twenty years. This isn't news to you. What may be news to you, however, is that the latest trends in bodybuilding nutrition have not only been questioning these standards but also have actually prescribed new plans that totally contradict them.

In fact, you could go so far as to say that in most bodybuilding circles nowadays, carbs are out and fats, yes FATS, are definitely in. In the past few years, a whole slew of bodybuilding and general fitness diets have sprung up that are high in protein and, in many cases, high in fat, while at the same time being extremely low in carbohydrates.

The reasoning and science behind these new programs goes something like this (at least in its condensed, simplified version). If you can shift the body away from burning glycogen (from carbohydrates) as its primary source of energy, it'll be forced to burn fat as fuel; thus, you'll burn not only the fat that you consume, but also any excess fat that's on your body.

A diet high in fat and low in carbohydrates forces your body to activate its fat burning enzymes (these are called lipolytic) while simultaneously decreasing its use of fat producing enzymes (lipogenic). The end result is that your body doesn't convert excess glucose into triglycerides (body fat). Instead, it burns the body fat you have while sparring the muscle building protein, and all is wonderful. That, at least, is the theory in a nutshell.

Some of you may recognize aspects of the Atkins' Diet that was popular in the 1970s and then again in the 1990s in all this. You're right. In fact, what seems like a new idea–high fat, low carbohydrate—has actually been around in some form or another for a very long time.

The most recent incarnation of this diet regimen has been sparked by programs like Protein Power and Dr. Barry Sears' Zone Diet plan. The Zone Diet, for instance, calls for dramatically reduced carbohydrate intake along with a necessary increase in the consumption of fats (though still mostly of the unsaturated variety). The Zone Diet is a program geared toward the general population, but the reasoning behind it has been applied more specifically to bodybuilding nutrition by numerous recent advocates and diet plans. Two in particular are worth mentioning.

The first of these is an interesting diet developed by Dr. Mario Depasquale. Dr. Depasquale's Anabolic Diet relies heavily on the theories of Atkins and Sears. Basically, it's a weekly cycle diet in which for the five days during the week you severely limit your carbohydrate intake to around 30 grams per day. That's not much . . . one apple and a half cup of yogurt and you're done with carbs for the day. No more carbs period. No bread, no pasta, no sugar, no rice, no milk, no cereal, no vegetables, no nothing when it comes to carbs.

You do eat a lot of fat and protein on these 5 days. The idea of course is to deplete your body of its glycogen stores and force it to burn fat for energy. Then for the two days on the weekend you eat anything you want. You name it, you can eat it. And believe me you will. This, of course, results in a type of rebound effect in which the body loads up on the carbohydrates. Theoretically producing a surge in growth hormones. The next week you repeat the cycle . . . and so on.

If you think that's rough, there's also the *Body Opus* diet by the late bodybuilding guru Dan Duchaine. The same patterns that you'll find in Atkins, Sears, and Dipasquale once again dominate, only this time they're taken to an almost masochistic extreme.

On the Body Opus Plan, for the 5 days during the week you aim to eat absolutely no carbohydrates . . . nada, none, zippo. Some carbs may slip in with other food, but you're shooting for absolute depletion. During those 5 days you eat 70% fat—that's right 70% fat—and 30% protein. As difficult as this sounds, the 70% fat is accomplished by eating lots of beef, whole eggs, pork, olive oil, cheese, bacon, sausage, and also supplementing with flaxseed oil.

On the weekends, you can eat some carbs, but still not as much as you're going to want. On these 2 days you should only up your calorie intake by about 20-25%. This Program is what's known as a ketogenic diet. The diet actually causes your body to be in a state of ketosis (generally not a good thing).

I definitely do not recommend this diet. The depravation is too extreme and could actually be hazardous to your health. Not to mention the fact that it's totally unnecessary. There are better, much less extreme ways to add lean muscle mass to your body without such drastic and dangerous nutritional techniques.

The mechanism at work in these diets—taking the body through cycles that produce a rebound anabolic effect–is valid. You see, it's really the carb loading phase of the programs, those two days on the weekend, that result in muscle growth.

I believe, in fact I know given my research and my experience, that this effect can be simulated in more subtle ways to produce even more dramatic long-term increases in muscle growth while simultaneously promoting overall health and well-being. In fact, the process actually *needs* to be done in a more subtle way in order to allow the body to train hard and preserve the muscle mass it gains.

The problem in general with these diet programs and others like them is their extremism. While it's true that you do have to push, prod, and cajole the body into adding muscle mass and/or losing fat, you don't have to push it to the edge of mental and physical breakdown. Again, I for one enjoy life too much to subject my body to these overly extreme measures.

There has to be and there is a better and a simpler way. It's called the *Anabolic Nutrition Program*, and it's the key to unlocking your body's natural capacity for muscle tissue production. Let me show you.

The Basics of the Anabolic Nutrition Program

Nutrient Sources: Compared with many of the other diet plans out there, this Program is not overly restrictive. There are times during your 4 week cycle, in fact, that you can eat almost anything you want (within the frequency and balance guidelines outlined below). In general, however, you'll want to stick with clean sources of whole foods.

For carbohydrates this means the bulk of your carbohydrate calories should come from complex carbs. You should be careful not to overdo it with simple sugars. Your post-workout drink is one notable exception to this general rule; more about this in a moment.

Try to get the bulk of your carbs from the complex food sources listed below:

NOT SO GOOD (EAT LESS)	BETTER (EAT MORE)	BEST (EAT MOST)
Glucose Honey Processed Sugars Soft Drinks Alcohol Most Cereals White Rice White Bread	Bananas Raisins White Spaghetti Flour Pancakes Brown Rice Whole Wheat Bread Potatoes	Oatmeal Sweet Potatoes Vegetables Fruits Wheat Spaghetti Wheat Pancakes Soy Beans Lentils Oats Fructose Kidney Beans

The list is necessarily incomplete or else we'd be here forever, but you get the idea. As much as you can, try to get the vast majority of your carbs from either the column on the right or the one in the center.

You'll need protein to support your new muscle growth. Some general rules apply to your protein intake as well. First of all, make sure you're getting about 1-1.5 grams of protein per pound of bodyweight per day. So if you weigh 180 lbs., you should shoot for around 180-270 grams of protein per day. Some experts will suggest slightly more or slightly less, but I've found this number works quite well and is easy to deal with.

In general, you'll want to concentrate on high-quality protein sources that aren't loaded with saturated fat. Here's a brief list of some of the basics and the amount of protein in a single 3 ½ oz serving:

SOURCE (3½ OZ)	PROTEIN (GRAMS)
Skinless Turkey Breast	23g
Skinless Chicken Breast	26g
Flounder	21g
Egg Whites	9g
Tuna (in water)	24g
Lean Beef	25g
Non-Fat Milk	3 ½g
Shrimp	17g
Salmon	20g

Another excellent and invaluable source of protein is protein powder. At roughly 20 grams of high-quality non-fat protein per serving, protein powders are a crucial supplement for those engaged in intense muscle training. Many companies are producing high-quality protein powders these days. Checkout the *Supplement Warehouse* at MuscleMaster.com for complete reviews and discount prices on all the latest products.

As far as fats are concerned, I'm a moderate. I feel that both a drastically low-fat diet (under 10%) or a drastically high-fat diet (over 30%) are counterproductive to lean muscle growth and building a first-rate physique. While it's OK to consume some saturated fat once in a while—I will not give up my occasional order of Buffalo Wings—you do need to distinguish between *good* fats and *bad* fats. And you do want the majority of the fats you consume to come from the *good* fats category.

HIGH IN BAD FATS	HIGH IN GOOD FATS
Peanut Oil	Flaxseed Oil
Coconut Oil	Canola Oil
Palm Oil	Virgin Olive Oil
Bacon Butter	Sunflower Oil
Pork Sausage	Shell Fish
Hamburger	Whole Eggs
Bologna	Salmon
Cheddar Cheese	Olives
Cream Cheese	Artichokes
Hot Dogs	Most Nuts/Seeds

The rule I've always used to distinguish the good from the bad when it comes to fats is that if it's loaded with grease—if you could sop it up with a paper towel—chances are it's loaded with bad or saturated fat. While saturated fat is not a total no, you should keep it to only about 10 % of your daily calorie intake if possible.

Meal Frequency: The scientific evidence is in: there's no doubt that to support the development of lean muscle mass you need to supply your body with a steady influx of nutrients. Ideally, this means that you should eat a well-balanced meal every three or four hours. That translates into 4-6 meals every day.

I am a great believer in the importance of frequent meals for muscle development, fat loss, and overall health, energy, and well-being. If there's one thing you can do to fuel your metabolism and change your body's composition, it's eat more frequently. If you're not eating at least 4 times a day (5 or 6 is even better), then you're not taking advantage of your body's natural processes and fueling your muscles to an optimum level.

Of course, your meals will be smaller than what the average person might consume at one sitting. The key is to space your nutrients out evenly over the course of the day, to keep your metabolism on high, and to constantly provide your growing muscles with the tissue-building nutrients they need.

I mention it in the *Ultimate Muscle Mass Training Program* and I'll mention it again here, when it comes to nutrition, timing is critical. For example, if you take two hypothetical people with the same exact genes and physical make-up, put them on the same training program, and have them eating the same 3000 calories per day, but person #1 is eating three 1000 calorie meals a day and person #2 is eating six 500 calorie meals a day, person #2 will ALWAYS have the better physique . . . period. More muscle, less fat.

The one thing you can do to immediately improve your nutrition and establish a base for muscle growth and fat lose is to eat frequent, well-balanced meals of roughly equal proportions.

Post-Workout Meal: Before we continue, a quick word about what you should eat immediately following a training session is necessary. Numerous studies have demonstrated the beneficial effects on muscle recovery and growth of a high carbohydrate, high protein meal immediately following an intense training session. These studies suggest that there exists a "window of opportunity" of approximately 60 minutes following your training in which the body can utilize extra carbs and protein very efficiently.

My own personal experiences with natural muscle development support these findings. You want to consume approximately 100 grams of carbohydrates within 30-60 minutes of the end of your training. You also want to take in about 30-40 grams of protein within about an hour.

Now if you're talking about solid food, that can translate into a pretty substantial meal. For many people, myself included, the digestive system won't respond too favorably to this type of meal right after an intense workout. It takes me a while before I feel really hungry. But you need to get those carbs and protein into your system quickly.

The solution is to use a carbohydrate replacement drink along with some protein powder or a meal replacement powder. This way, your body gets the nutrients that your muscles immediately need in a way that you and your digestive system can handle.

Calorie Distribution: So you now have some general rules about carbohydrates, proteins, and fats that you need to be aware of and keep in mind. And you also understand the importance of the post-workout meal. The next area to pin down is how much of each nutrient you want to consume on average to maximize your body's anabolic processes and fuel your intense training. In other words, what's the best nutrient distribution to ensure that your muscles will grow.

While individual needs will always vary slightly, you want to start with a base distribution of 50-30-20 and then adjust it accordingly depending on what stage of the 4 Week anabolic cycle you're in. More about this in a moment.

Your base nutrient distribution then calls for you to get approximately 50% of your daily calories from carbohydrates (emphasizing complex forms); 30% of your calories will come from quality protein sources; and 20% of your calories will come from fats with no more than half that, or 10%, from saturated fats.

These numbers may be slightly higher in total fats and slightly lower in total carbohydrates then you're used to. Not only is that OK, it's actually a necessary step to allow for optimized muscle development. And don't worry, the extra fat calories will not translate into extra fat (an all too common misconception) provided that you follow the program through all 4 Weeks of the cycle.

Establishing Your Baselines: As I mentioned before, I'm not an obsessive calorie counter, and this nutrition program isn't about that. But while it's not necessary to tally up every last calorie, it is necessary to at least have some estimates to work with in developing your individualized plan. Not everyone, after all, is starting at the same point in their training or, for that matter, at the same bodyweight.

One thing you'll need to have is an estimate of your daily maintenance level calorie requirements. How many calories, in other words, do you need to consume daily to maintain your current bodyweight given your current level of activity?

Many of you will already have a pretty good idea of what your daily maintenance number is. If you don't, there are several ways to calculate it, though none of them are individualized enough to be universally valid. These methods, however, will provide you with some estimates that should be sufficient for our purposes.

Maybe the most individually accurate but also the most time-consuming way to calculate your maintenance level calorie requirements is to keep track of your total calorie intake over the course of 5 average days; these are days where you don't gain or lose a significant amount of weight. You should note that 2 lbs. or 3 lbs. either way is insignificant because of natural fluctuations in fluid levels.

Add up all your calories for the 5 days and divide that number by 5. While certainly not flawless, this should give you a pretty good number to work with, and it will be significantly more accurate than if you only tracked one or two days.

A less time consuming method that will enable you to come up with a decent estimate of your maintenance level calorie requirements is to do the following calculations:

Step 1

Multiply your weight in pounds by 13.8: _____
Add your height in inches multiplied by 5:   + _____
Add the following number: +   66.5
Total: = _____
Now subtract your age in years multiplied by 6.8: - _____
Total: = _____

Step 2

Take the number you calculated above: _____

Add 5% of this number to it if you are inactive;
Add 10% of this number to it if you are moderately active;
Add 15% of this number to it if you are active.
Add 20% of this number to it if you are extremely active.

Estimated Total Maintenance Daily Calorie Requirements: _____

One final way to calculate your total maintenance daily calorie requirements is extremely simple. Just take your weight in pounds and multiply it by 18 if you are currently training intensely. Multiply your weight by 14 if you only exercise moderately.

You can do both Method #2 and Method #3 relatively quickly and compare results.

Let's use as an example a 25 year old who weighs 180 lbs., is 6 ft tall, and is actively training. Using the second method, the maintenance calorie requirement for this individual would be roughly 3290. If we use the third method (180 x 18) the total comes out to 3240. Either way, the totals are pretty close: in the 3200-3300 range. This is the type of estimate we need.

Now the next step is to apply your total *Maintenance* daily calorie requirements to the 50-30-20 carb, protein, fat base calorie distribution ratio.

Let's use the same example from above and take the 3200 number to make it easy. Our hypothetical 180 lbs. individual should shoot for 50% of his calories from carbohydrates (1600), 30% from proteins (960), and 20% from fats (640).

Now calculate your base calorie distribution ratios:

Take your **Total Daily Maintenance Calorie Requirements:** _____
Multiply by 50% (.50) for your total daily carbohydrate base: _____
Multiply by 30% (.30) for your total daily protein base: _____
Multiply by 20% (.20) for your total daily fat base: _____

We can now carry the calculations one-step further to determine the base total for carbohydrates, proteins, and fats in terms of grams. All you need to know is that 1 gram of carbs = 4 calories; 1 gram of protein = 4 calories; and 1 gram of fat = 9 calories.

To calculate your gram requirements you simply divide the individual totals for carbs by 4, for proteins by 4, and for fats by 9. Let's use our example again.

Carbohydrates: 1600 ÷ 4 = 400 grams
Proteins: 960 ÷ 4 = 240 grams
Fats: 640 ÷ 9 = 71 grams

Now calculate your own base daily gram targets for each of the following:

Carbohydrates: _____ ÷ 4 = _____ grams
Proteins: _____ ÷ 4 = _____ grams
Fats: _____ ÷ 9 = _____ grams

Again, these numbers aren't absolutes. You just want to have some idea of where your baseline is so you're not totally in the dark about your nutrient requirements and how they break down into grams.

Establishing Your Per Meal Baselines: Now that you've determined your *Maintenance* baselines for daily total calories, carbohydrate calories, protein calories, and fat calories—as well as the total gram equivalents for each of these three calorie sources—the next crucial step is geared towards making your life a whole lot easier.

At this point, you want to calculate your per meal requirements. You see, it's always much easier to break things down into their simplest units. It's easier, in other words, to think about what nutrients you have to get in each meal than to worry about total daily intake.

You do this simply by dividing your totals by the number of meals you can get in each day on average. As I mentioned above, you need to get at least 4 and hopefully 6 meals in every day. Since I believe 6 is the optimum number, I'll apply it to my example. I always find it easier to deal with grams than calories, so estimating I'd break it down like this:

Per Meal Targets:

    Carbohydrates: 400 grams ÷ 6 = 67 grams/meal
    Proteins: 240 grams ÷ 6 = 40 grams/meal
    Fats: 71 grams ÷ 6 = 12 grams/meal

Now plug in your baseline numbers:

Per Meal Targets:

    Carbohydrates: ____ grams ÷ __ = ____ grams/meal
    Proteins: ____ grams ÷ __ = ____ grams/meal
    Fats: ____ grams ÷ __ = ____ grams/meal

These then are your *Maintenance* level targets for each meal. Obviously you're not going to have meals that are always right on the money, but once you've worked with your Plan for a month or so, you actually develop a repertoire of meals that come very close to your targets. Soon you'll also begin to develop an instinct for knowing how much to eat with any given meal. It really becomes almost second nature.

But remember, this is only your baseline for *Maintenance* level nutrient intake. Your goal is to add muscle, not to stay where you are. To do so, you're going to need to use the knowledge you've gained about your requirements and apply it to a systematic program aimed at pushing your body to new levels of muscle growth.

The Principle of Variation: As with your muscle training itself, when it comes to your diet variation is once again the key element in producing significant muscle growth. You see, if you eat the same amounts of the same nutrients all the time, your body will do what it does best: it will adjust to this level of intake and once accustomed to it will stop changing. In this case, it'll stop growing. We need, therefore, to take some very deliberate measures to avoid this.

Incidentally, the body's inherent ability to adjust is precisely why most of the traditional weight gain or weight lose diets will work for a short period of time and then stop working altogether. They work when you first try them because they represent a shock or at least a new stimulus to the body. They stop working because the body eventually adjusts to them and compensates.

Any nutrition program that hopes to achieve continual muscle building results over the long haul must have significant variation built into it. Make no mistake about it. Variety is not only the spice of life, it's the driving force behind continual muscle growth.

The trick is to develop a nutrition program that uses the muscle building power of variation while at the same time remaining relatively easy to follow and apply. The best solution that I've discovered is a simple 4 Week repeating cycle.

The Anabolic Nutrition Program

The *Anabolic Nutrition Program* is based on a repeating 4 Week Cycle and the following three distinct patterns of nutrient consumption:

1. Maintenance Level Calorie and Nutrient Consumption;
2. Restricted or Low Level Calorie and Nutrient Consumption;
3. Super-Compensation or High Level Calorie and Nutrient Consumption.

The Program works because it does not allow the body to adapt to a consistent pattern of calorie and nutrient intake. There is, in other words, enough variation built into the diet that the body is placed in a fairly constant state of flux.

The result of this carefully constructed variation is a dramatic elevation in the amount of natural anabolic hormones released during the *Super-Compensation* phase; this, of course, translates into dramatic muscle growth.

It's important to stress that it's not the *Super-Compensation* phase in and of itself that produces the anabolic increases in the body and the resulting increases in lean muscle tissue. If it was, we could just eat a high calorie diet all the time. Rather, it is the unique combination of all three phases of the Program which result in producing a biological and chemical condition in the body that is particularly conducive to increased muscle growth.

It's the variation along with the timing and the structuring of the three individual diet phases which leads to muscle growth. This is the key. When I discovered the anabolic importance of phasing nutrient consumption after years of research and experimentation with my own diet, it seemed so obvious and so simple.

Bodybuilders have traditionally gone through long periods of over-eating during their bulking phases and long, difficult, and in some cases dangerous periods of calorie deprivation during their cutting phases. This is not a good idea. After just a few weeks, the body is able to adjust to any diet and progress, whether you're trying to gain weight in the form of lean muscle mass or to lose weight in the form of body fat, will slow significantly and may eventually come to a halt altogether.

We haven't even mentioned how tedious and boring any fixed diet (as opposed to one based on variation) can quickly become. *The Anabolic Nutrition Program* solves these and many other problems because your nutrient intake changes significantly three times during every 4 Week Cycle. Nevertheless, these crucial changes are simple and understandable enough for all of us to easily implement without becoming obsessed with our diets.

Because each of us is starting from different points–some have been restricting their diet for a while, others have paid little attention to what they eat—and also because it's important to begin the Program with the body in a state of normalcy, the *Anabolic Nutrition Program* begins with one week (a full 7 days) of *Maintenance* level calorie and micronutrient consumption.

This is immediately followed by one week of *Restricted* or low level calorie and micronutrient consumption to prime the body for the upcoming rush of anabolic, growth-producing hormones.

After this one week *Restricted* calorie consumption phase, we immediately shift to the *Super-Compensation* or high level calorie and micronutrient consumption phase. Doing so actually shocks the body into releasing extra levels of insulin, growth hormone, testosterone, and other natural anabolic substances.

Because we are interested in adding muscle mass, and because the scientific evidence suggests that this period of increased anabolism can last up to 14 days, the *Super-Compensation* phase of the cycle lasts a full two weeks.

The 4 Week Cycle can be repeated–provided that the duration of each mini-cycle and the order of the weeks stays the same—until the desired level of muscle mass is reached.

Because variation is built into the Program, the body will not adjust to this 4 Week Cycle; you'll continue to see results until you reach the genetic limits of your muscle building potential. For most average height natural bodybuilders with average genetics, I've found that this limit is somewhere around 220 lbs. (give or take 10 lbs. or so) of bodyweight with around 5% to 8% body fat.

While individual results will always vary, most individuals using this Program and training intensely with sufficient recovery time can expect to gain 2-6 lbs. of lean body mass at the conclusion of each 4 Week Cycle. As anyone who's been training for a while will know, this is a significant, even extraordinary, amount of muscle to gain in such a short period of time. The key is the Principle of Variation, and what follows are the details of how you put that principle into practice.

WEEK 1: Maintenance Level Calorie and Nutrient Phase

You begin the Program with a full week at your *Maintenance* level diet. As always, you should be eating at least 4 and preferably 5 or 6 balanced and roughly equal meals throughout the day.

One way of getting all those meals in is to use some key supplements; in particular, you will find Meal Replacement Powders (MRPs) to be invaluable. Make them an integral part of your everyday nutritional plan. You've probably seen these instant meals in an envelope by now. They're put out by many different companies. These MRPs, as they're called, are generally high in protein, low in fat, and low to moderate in carbohydrates. They mix up well with water, juice, or milk.

I use MRPs a lot. They can really come in handy when you're trying to get five or six quality meals in a day. If you're like me, you won't have much time to prepare all those meals, but with MRPs all you need to do is open the envelope and mix it up. Plus you can take them anywhere you go. I suggest you get one, two, or even three of your meals each day in this way. Visit the *Supplement Warehouse* at MuscleMaster.com for specific recommendations and product discounts.

Remember, for this week you're simply going to work with your *Maintenance* daily calorie and nutrient requirements—the one that you calculated earlier. When you've divided the total by the number of meals you're able to get in, you'll have your target numbers for every day and every meal this week.

Let's take the example of the 180 lbs. individual that we used before. Using the 50-30-20 breakdown, here are the approximate daily targets we worked out:

Calories:	3200
Carbohydrates:	400 grams
Proteins:	240 grams
Fats:	71 grams

And assuming a total of 6 meals each day, these are the approximate per meal targets:

Calories	530
Carbohydrates:	67 grams
Proteins:	40 grams
Fats:	12 grams

It's important to reiterate at this point that these are simply approximate targets; as long as you're in the general range, you're on track. When push comes to shove, the most important element in the equation is the total calories. This individual wants to be around 500-550 calories per meal. He doesn't want to eat a meal with only 200 calories, and he certainly doesn't want to be consistently eating 1000 calorie meals this week.

For me, all of the per meal targets are pretty easy to manage with the occasional exception of the protein, which can sometimes be more challenging. This is where a high-quality protein powder becomes helpful. I can mix up a quick scoop with some water, milk or juice to get me to my target numbers.

Once you've got your *Maintenance* targets down, you'll find it very useful to develop a basic repertoire of 10-12 meals which you can draw from. Incidentally, I often use the same meals during the *Restricted* and the *Super-Compensation* phases of the Program. I simply adjust the portions down or up as the case may be. It really does become a very easy Program to follow once you're accustomed to it.

Since everyone's targets will be different, everyone's meals will also necessarily be highly individualized. But here are a few examples of *Maintenance* level meals that I would suggest for our hypothetical 180 lbs. weight trainer:

SAMPLE MEAL #1	SAMPLE MEAL #2	SAMPLE MEAL #3
Omelet (2 whole eggs, 4 egg whites, 2oz mushrooms), 2 Slices Whole Grain Toast, Apple	Meal Replacement Powder, ¼ Cup Brown Rice (sprinkled with Olive Oil)	Skinless Chicken Breast (3 oz) cooked with garlic and Olive Oil, 2 Sweet potatoes, 2 Cups Broccoli
Calories: 540 Carbs: 75 grams Protein: 38 grams Fat: 10 grams	Calories: 540 Carbs: 64 grams Protein: 40 grams Fat: 14 grams	Calories: 500 Carbs: 70 grams Protein: 36 grams Fat: 12 grams

Again, as much as possible, all of your meals should be structured in a similar way this week: a way that reflects your *Maintenance* level calorie requirements and our basic 50-30-20 carbohydrate, protein, fat ratio.

Once you get into the swing of it, you'll find out what you like and what you need to have around your kitchen to meet your targets. I already mentioned the importance of protein powder. Some of my other favorite tricks to help me hit the targets include cooking up a batch of chicken breasts or other lean meat so I have 4-5 days supply readily at hand. I also like to do this with my brown rice and whole grain pasta. I find I use a lot of oatmeal, and of course Olive Oil and/or Flaxseed Oil is a must.

Food prep really does become second nature once you get the hang of the Program. It's just a matter of combining the right foods and using your supplements wisely throughout the day. Again, you should be eating every 3-4 hours to keep your body fueled and in a positive nitrogen balance to promote general health as well as muscle development.

During this first week, your training should be of moderate intensity. This and other important training guidelines are outlined in full detail in the *Ultimate Muscle Mass Training Program* I've developed.

WEEK 2: Restricted or Low Level Calorie and Nutrient Phase

For many of us, this may be the most difficult week in the cycle . . . it may also be the most important. This is the week where you must prime your body for the anabolic growth period that will follow. In order to successfully do this, you must restrict your overall calorie intake significantly.

You see, you want to put your body into a temporary state of calorie and nutrient deprivation. I emphasize the word *temporary* here. You need to understand that this is a necessary step in this 3-step process. The ultimate goal of adding a significant amount of muscle mass to your frame will only be optimized if your body is jolted into an anabolic state. The *Restricted* calorie phase of the cycle is what allows that jolt to take place.

At this point, you should not be concerned that you will lose weight or muscle mass during this brief period. The scientific evidence is conclusive that if you do lose some weight, nearly all of it will be from body fat, the muscle will be preserved, and the pound or two that you may drop will quickly be added back, and then some, once you enter the *Super-Compensation* phase of the cycle. But without the *Restricted* calorie phase, there can be no *Super-Compensation* phase, and you won't ultimately be adding the type of muscle mass you desire.

During the 7 day period of the *Restricted* phase, you want to cut your overall calorie intake in half. You still want to eat 4-6 evenly spaced meals per day, but they'll need to be small meals—each one about half the size of those in your *Maintenance* diet. You want to cut the bulk of your calories from carbohydrates and fats. You should keep your protein intake relatively high to help preserve your muscle mass.

Your calorie distribution this week should be in the 40-50-10 range. So now you'll be shooting to get 40% of your calories from carbohydrates; a full 50% from proteins; and only 10% from fats. When you factor in that you'll be consuming only about half your *Maintenance* daily calories, you'll be restricting your carbohydrate intake quite substantially. You'll still be well within the safe carbohydrate range, however, and ketosis will not be a problem.

Here's what the daily calorie and nutrient targets would look like this week for our 180 lbs. trainer (reflecting the 40-50-10 breakdown):

Calories:	1600
Carbohydrates:	160 grams
Proteins:	200 grams
Fats:	18 grams

And assuming a total of 6 meals each day, these are the approximate per meal targets:

Calories	270
Carbohydrates:	26 grams
Proteins:	33 grams
Fats:	3 grams

At this point, you should figure out your own target estimates for this week. First do your daily targets:

Take Your Maintenance Level Daily Calories: _____
Divide by 2 for your Restricted Calorie Total: _____
Multiply line #2 by 40% (.40): _____
Divide by 4 for your Daily Carbohydrate Target: _____ grams
Multiply line #2 by 50% (.50): _____
Divide by 4 for your Daily Protein Target: _____ grams
Multiply line #2 by 10% (.10): _____
Divide by 9 for your Daily Fat Target: _____ grams

Now divide lines #1, #4, #6, and #8 by the total number of meals you can get in each day to get your per meal targets. Record your *Restricted* per meal targets here:

Calories	_____	
Carbohydrates:	_____	grams
Proteins:	_____	grams
Fats:	_____	grams

You'll likely feel pretty hungry during the week, especially the first day or two. This is normal; it's basically the price you have to pay to get the anabolic explosion you're looking for in the next two weeks. If you make sure you eat a little bit every three hours or so, you'll alleviate a lot of the pangs and make things a bit easier on yourself.

If you are already relatively lean, then one of the added benefits of this week is that your body will basically strip off any excess fat you might have hanging around—your abs should come out a bit more than usual, and your muscles will look ripped.

Be sure to drink plenty of water this week . . . you should, of course, be doing this all the time any way. Also, keep your training intensity down pretty low during these *Restricted* calorie periods. We're preparing our bodies to build muscle at this point; we're not there yet. Another quick note: those Meal Replacement Powders come in particularly handy this week because they're high in protein and low in carbohydrates and fat. I use them for up to three or even four meals a day during the *Restricted* calorie phase.

Be sure to maintain this *Restricted* calorie and nutrient intake for the full seven days. The big pay-off in significant new muscle mass is about to happen.

WEEKS 3 & 4: Super-Compensation or High Calorie and Nutrient Phase

Get ready to explode! The Restricted phase you've just struggled through is about to pay-off big time. At this point, your body is now primed and ready to be jolted into an extended anabolic period.

During this period, you still stick with your 4-6 meals per day schedule, only now instead of subtracting from your *Maintenance* level targets, you add to them. And you add to them substantially. Your body and your appetite should be primed and ready to eat in a serious way. Your job during these two key weeks is to accommodate them.

The goal here is to up your daily calorie intake by about 50% for the full 14 days. So our 180 lbs. trainer with a *Maintenance* daily requirement of 3200 calories would go up to about 4800 calories total per day. You should figure out your *Super-Compensation* daily calorie target here:

       Take your Maintenance level calorie base: _____
       Divide by 2 = _____
       Add lines #1 and #2 together for your total: _____

Again, this is an estimate that you should shoot for. The most important thing during this two week period is that you eat a lot. That's really the bottom line.

You see, it's well known that food is in and of itself an anabolic catalyst. If you're training hard, eating a substantial amount of food sets into motion an entire series of anabolic processes in the body. Hormones are released, and the release of insulin and growth hormone in particular seems to contribute extensively to the development of muscle mass in individuals involved with intense resistance training.

By going through the *Restricted* calorie phase of the cycle, you've basically fired your body up to rebound in this *Super-Compensation* phase with the maximum amounts of muscle producing hormones that it can. It's almost as if you've put a temporary dam up to hold back the surge of anabolic hormones in your body; once the dam breaks or is lifted, the anabolic waters come surging forward with ten times their original force. This is the mechanism behind the entire *Anabolic Nutrition Program*.

So the *Super-Compensation* phase causes this tremendous surge in an all-natural anabolic state; it's still only a temporary surge, but it's one you can maintain for up to two full weeks. After that, your body is up to its old tricks of adjusting and adapting to the situation at hand. At that point, it's once again time to change things up. For now though, it's time to eat and to train with extremely high intensity. You want to train with great focus and effort to capitalize on the anabolic surge that your diet cycling has caused.

To reiterate, during the *Super-Compensation* phase calories are the most important consideration. You can basically eat as much clean, healthy food as you want, though you still should have 4-6 relatively equal size meals per day. You can splurge a bit and include some cheat foods during this period.

Our hypothetical 180 lbs. trainer would want to be around 800 calories per meal (4800 ÷ 6 = 800) during these two weeks. You should calculate your target calories per meal so that you have a rough idea of what you're shooting for:

Total Daily Calories during Super-Compensation Phase: _____
Total Meals per Day: ÷ _____
Average Calories per Meal: _____

If you'd like to break it down into the nutrient components you can, although it isn't absolutely necessary to do so during this Phase. The ideal breakdown would be a bit different than the prior ones we've calculated. During *Super-Compensation* you actually want extra carbohydrates because of their insulin-releasing attributes.

The breakdown I've had the most success with here is 60-20-20 where 60% of your daily calories come from carbohydrates; 20% from proteins: and 20% from fats. The end result of these new ratios is that during this 2 week growth period you're getting a lot more carbohydrates than usual and a bit more fat (which can also act as an anabolic stimulant). Your protein intake, on the other hand, stays fairly consistent throughout.

Let's apply this new 60-20-20 ratio to our hypothetical trainer so you can see what I mean. His daily targets would breakdown like this:

    Calories: 4800
    Carbohydrates: 720 grams
    Proteins: 240 grams
    Fats: 106 grams

You'll notice in particular how significantly carbohydrate intake has shot up. This is exactly what we want—carbs are the key to getting the body to release the anabolic cocktail we're after. Fat intake too can go up a bit from your *Maintenance* level. Go ahead and have that cheeseburger or Mexican food you love during these two weeks. Don't worry about adding a lot of excess fat; your body isn't interested in this . . . it's in an anabolic muscle building state! Though protein intake as a percentage of total calories drops from your *Maintenance* level (from 30% down to 20%), actual intake in terms of grams pretty much holds steady (in this case 240 grams).

If you want, we can carry the breakdowns through to the next step by calculating per meal targets as we did previously. Our sample trainer's per meal targets during this *Super-Compensation* phase—assuming the usual 6 meals per day—would look something like this:

Calories:	800
Carbohydrates:	120 grams
Proteins:	40 grams
Fats:	18 grams

That's quite a bit of food, but it's what is required if you are going to shock your body into some serious new muscle growth.

Keeping in mind that these targets during the *Super-Compensation* phase are really the loosest guidelines of any of the three Phases, go ahead and calculate your own targets to at least get a sense of where they're at. Start with your daily targets:

Take Your Super-Compensation Level Daily Calories:	_____	
Multiply line #1 by 60% (.60):	_____	
Divide by 4 for your Daily Carbohydrate Target:	_____	grams
Multiply line #1 by 20% (.20):	_____	
Divide by 4 for your Daily Protein Target:	_____	grams
Multiply line #1 by 20% (.20):	_____	
Divide by 9 for your Daily Fat Target:	_____	grams

Now divide lines #1, #3, #5, and #7 by the total number of meals you can get in each day to get your per meal targets. Record your *Super-Compensation* per meal targets here:

        Calories   _____
        Carbohydrates: _____ grams
        Proteins: _____ grams
        Fats: _____ grams

At this point, you should have some general targets down on paper for each of the Three Phases of the Program. Remember, this isn't a math exam; you don't have to weigh and calculate everything out every day to make the *Anabolic Nutrition Program* work. As long as your in the target range, you'll be accomplishing what you need to place your body into an anabolic state and stimulate new lean muscle mass.

Needless to say, it's during this *Super-Compensation* two week period of the four week Cycle that you should train the hardest and eat the most. You'll feel strong and pumped due to the rapid introduction of extra nutrients into your body. And you should take advantage of that strength by really pushing yourself in the gym. In fact, if you're manipulating your diet properly, this 2 week phase of the cycle will produce almost a drug-like effect on you and your physique . . . and it's totally natural!

Once the two weeks are up, it's important not to continue the *Super-Compensation* phase of the Program any longer. You see, after about 14 days your body will do its thing, adapt to the situation, and start using those extra calories to store fat rather than to build muscle. That's something we certainly don't want.

You've got your 14 day window of opportunity to add some significant muscle mass; eat up, but after that period has passed, you need to return to Week 1 of the Cycle and start over again.

As I said earlier, you can continue to successfully use this 4 Week Cycle over and over again indefinitely. Variation is built into it, so your body simply won't be able to adapt in any lasting way before you're once again shifting into a drastically different phase of the Program.

When you repeat the 4 Week Cycle, however, there is one very important consideration that you have to be aware of. It seems obvious, but many people forget that when they start their second or third cycle they may be 5 lbs. or even 10 lbs. heavier in terms of lean muscle mass than when they began their first. If you're 5 lbs. or 10 lbs. heavier—you guessed it—your daily calorie and nutrient requirements are going to be higher during every Phase of the Program. You'll need to recalculate your *Maintenance, Restriction,* and *Super-Compensation* daily targets. Believe me, it's a small price to pay for the type of quality muscle mass that you'll pack on as a result of this attention to detail.

Some Final Thoughts

Finally, let me just reiterate as I always do that I hope this is just the beginning of our journey together. I hope you'll keep me informed about your progress, and I invite you to stay in touch.

I hope too that this *Anabolic Nutrition Program* works as well for you as it has for me and the ever-growing number of people who are using it to look and feel their best. The Program was born out of necessity, out of my own individual frustration with and confusion about the myriad of diets and nutrition plans available.

In searching for a simple and workable plan that I could use to naturally and safely add muscle mass, I've discovered that the anabolic potential of the human body is simply remarkable. I've learned too that the capacity to transform our physiques, to add significant and lasting muscle, exists within us all.

Your job is to simply tap into the muscle building capability within yourself . . . to be your best . . . and to enjoy the ride. Good Luck!